DOG FOOD RECIPES COOKBOOK:

Barking Delights, Tempting Homemade Recipes Tailored for Dogs

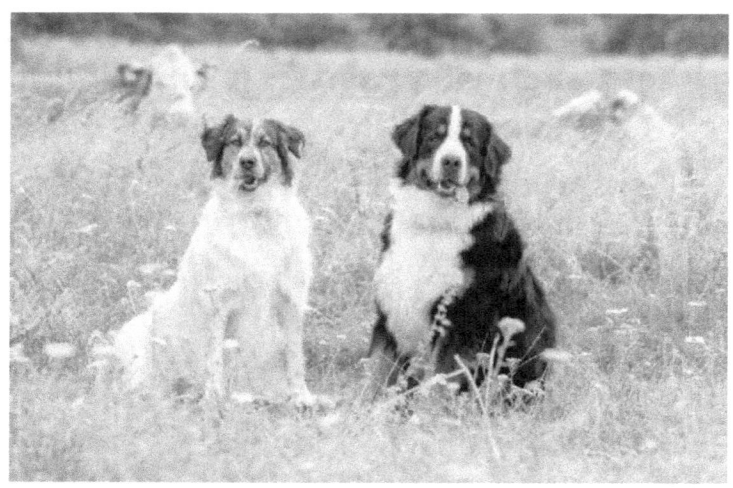

Elsa Treece

Chapter 1: Introduction

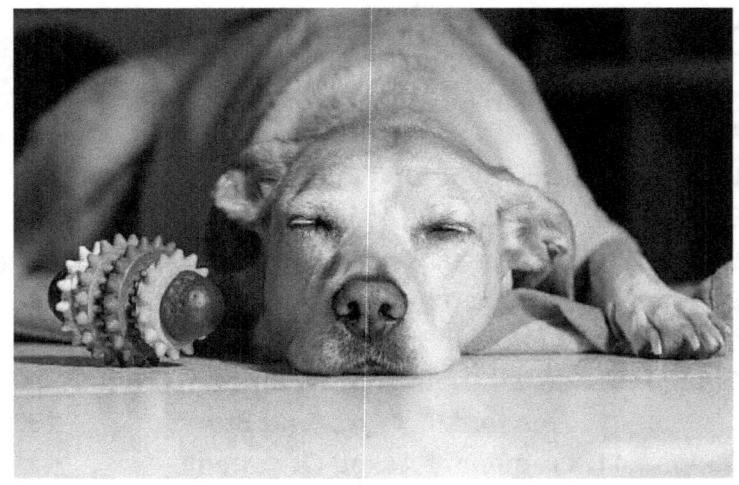

1.1 About This Cookbook

Welcome to the Canine Food Recipes Cookbook! The goal of this cookbook is to provide you with a collection of healthy and delicious dishes that you can make at home for your pet. Dogs enjoy tasty meals, and if you make their food yourself, you can ensure that it contains only high-quality, wholesome ingredients and no unnecessary additives.

In this cookbook, you'll find various recipes sorted into various segments, including meat-based recipes, fish-based recipes, veggie lover and vegetarian choices, as well as treats and bites. We have likewise remembered a part of extraordinary eating regimens and well-being concerns, offering recipes customized for canines with explicit dietary necessities or medical issues.

By setting up your canine's dinners at home, you have the valuable chance to assume command over their sustenance and take special care of their singular requirements. You'll discover how enjoyable it is to cook for your pet and how satisfying it is to provide them with a well-balanced and flavorful diet.

Before jumping into the recipes, it's vital to comprehend the rudiments of canine sustenance and the fundamental supplements canines expect to flourish.

We'll walk you through these fundamentals so you can choose the right ingredients and cook your dog's meals with confidence.

Furthermore, we'll give you tips on kitchen fundamentals for canine food arrangement, including the devices and gear you'll require, as well as direction on segment control and taking care of rules. We'll likewise resolve normal various forms of feedback you might have about changing to natively constructed canine food and the well-being contemplations to remember.

Whether you're hoping to change your canine to a hand-crafted diet or essentially need to integrate a few custom-made feasts and treats into their daily schedule, this cookbook is your go-to asset. So we should begin on this intriguing culinary excursion, making delectable feasts that will make your shaggy companion's tail sway with enchantment!

1.2 Benefits of Homemade Dog Food

Taking care of your canine's hand-crafted food offers a few advantages that add to their general well-being and prosperity. The following are some significant advantages of feeding homemade dog food to your pet:

1.   Oversight of the Ingredients: You have complete control over the ingredients when you cook dog food at home. You can pick top-notch meats, new leafy foods, and entire grains, guaranteeing that your canine gets nourishment from healthy sources. If your dog has particular allergies or dietary restrictions, this control is especially useful.

2.   Preservatives and additives should be avoided: Business canine food sources frequently contain added substances, additives, and counterfeit flavors that may not be great for your canine's well-being. You can get rid of these additives by making

homemade meals for your dog, giving him a diet that is more natural and full of nutrients.

3. Personalized Diet: Each canine is remarkable, with various wholesome requirements in light of variables, for example, age, breed, action level, and ailments. Hand-crafted canine food permits you to alter your canine's feasts to meet their particular prerequisites. You can change segment sizes, balance macronutrients, and integrate supplements depending on the situation to guarantee a balanced and adjusted diet.

4. Expanded Absorbability: A few canines might have responsive qualities or stomach-related issues that can be mitigated by changing to natively constructed food. With painstakingly chosen fixings and appropriate cooking techniques, you can make dinners that are all the more effectively edible for your shaggy

companion, diminishing the gamble of gastrointestinal inconvenience.

5.   Improved Tastefulness: Canines are many times more excited about hand-crafted feasts because of their upgraded flavor and fragrance. You can make tasty meals that your dog will love by experimenting with different seasonings and ingredients. This will encourage your dog to eat well and enjoy mealtimes.

6.   Engagement and connection: Getting ready for custom-made canine food permits you to partake in your canine's nourishment and care effectively. It tends to be a remunerating experience that fortifies the connection between you and your shaggy friend. Including your canine in the cooking system or evaluating custom-made treats together can be a tomfoolery and intuitive method for investing quality energy.

Although making your dog food has many advantages, you must approach it carefully and with knowledge. Talk with your veterinarian or a veterinary nutritionist to guarantee that your canine's dietary necessities are being met. They can give direction on segment sizes, explicit supplement prerequisites, and any changes required given your canine's singular conditions.

Keep in mind, custom-made canine food ought to be ready with thoughtfulness regarding cleanliness, legitimate food taken care of, and adjusted nourishment. Homemade meals can be a wonderful addition to your dog's diet, promoting their health and happiness, if you prepare them properly and pay attention to their well-being.

1.3 Safety Considerations

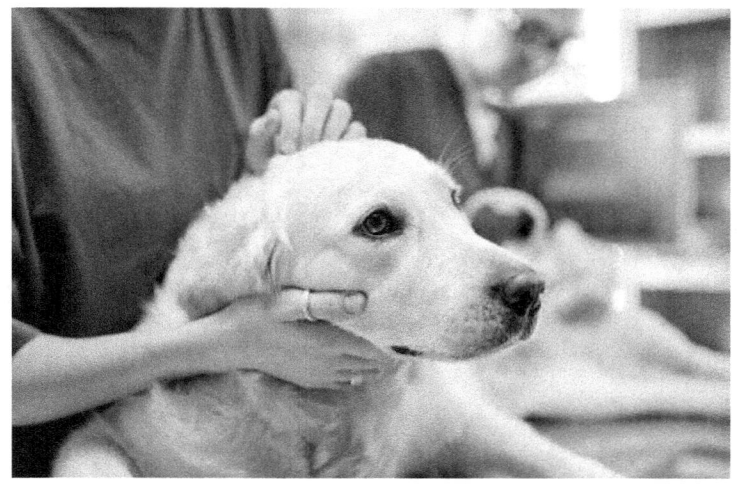

While getting ready for natively constructed canine food offers many advantages, focusing on your canine's security and prosperity is significant. When making homemade dog food, the following essential safety considerations should be kept in mind:

1.   Talk with a Veterinarian: Consultation with a veterinarian or veterinary nutritionist is essential before making any significant dietary adjustments for your dog. They can help you create a balanced diet that is tailored to your dog's needs, offer guidance

on ingredient selection, and provide valuable insights into the specific nutritional requirements of your dog.

2. Wholesome Equilibrium: Dogs require a well-balanced diet rich in vitamins, minerals, protein, carbohydrates, and healthy fats. Guarantee that your hand-crafted canine food recipes give a legitimate equilibrium of these fundamental supplements. A nutritionist can assist you with working out the proper proportions and guide you on any important enhancements.

3. Stay away from Unsafe Fixings: Dogs may be harmed or poisoned by certain human foods. Stay away from fixings like chocolate, onions, garlic, grapes, raisins, avocados, and certain counterfeit sugars like xylitol. Research and get to know food sources that ought to have stayed away from to forestall potential well-being takes a chance for your canine.

4. Using food safely: Pursue great sanitation routines while getting ready custom-made canine food. Before and after handling raw ingredients, thoroughly wash your hands and make sure all utensils, bowls, and surfaces are clean. To avoid cross-contamination, keep raw meats separate from other ingredients and immediately freeze or refrigerate leftovers.

5. Quality Fixings: Make sure the ingredients in your dog's food are of high quality. Pick lean meats, new products of the soil, and entire grains. Try not to utilize fixings that are past their lapse date or have been put away inappropriately. Quality fixings add to the healthy benefit and in general security of the food you plan.

6. Sensitivities and Awarenesses: Very much like people, canines can have sensitivities or aversions to specific food varieties. Be on the lookout for your dog's

reactions to new ingredients and any indications of digestive problems, itching, or other allergic reactions. Assuming you suspect a sensitivity or responsiveness, talk with your veterinarian for proper testing and direction.

7. Segment Control: Overloading can prompt weight gain and related medical problems. Observe segment rules given by your veterinarian or nutritionist in light of your canine's age, breed, weight, and movement level. Consistently screen your canine's weight and change segment sizes on a case-by-case basis to keep a sound weight.

8. Slow Change: If you're switching your dog's diet from store-bought to homemade, do so gradually to avoid gastrointestinal problems. Steadily present new fixings and change proportions throughout possibly 14 days, permitting your canine's stomach-related framework to adjust to the changes.

You can ensure that your homemade dog food is not only nutritious but also safe for your pet by considering these safety precautions. When preparing your dog's meals, the health and well-being of your dog should always come first. Experts can be of great assistance throughout the process.

Chapter 2: Dog Nutrition Basics

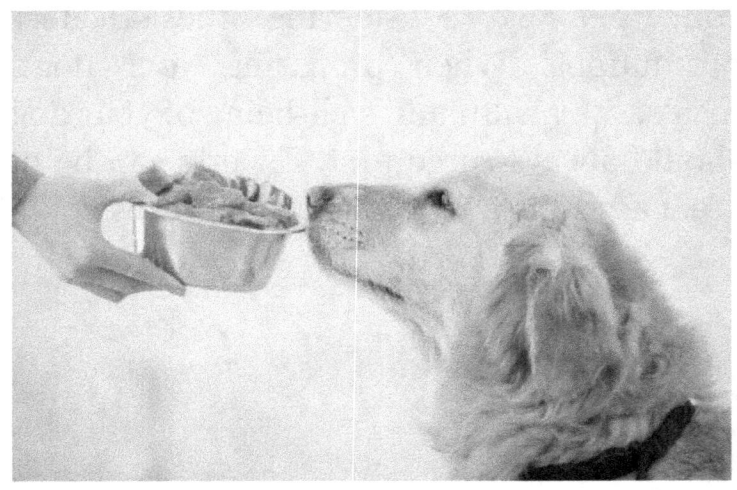

2.1 Understanding Your Dog's Nutritional Needs

To give your canine a solid and adjusted custom-made diet, understanding their wholesome needs is fundamental. Canines require explicit supplements to help their development, energy levels, and general prosperity. Here are a few critical elements to consider while planning custom-made canine food:

1.   Protein: Your dog needs a lot of protein in his diet. It encourages muscle growth, tissue repair, and overall wellness. For vegetarian or vegan diets, lean meats like chicken, beef, turkey, or fish, eggs, and plant-based proteins like legumes or tofu are good sources of protein for dogs. When incorporating both animal and plant-based proteins, try to achieve a balance.

2.   Carbohydrates: Sugars give energy and fiber to your canine's eating routine. Pick complex starches like earthy-colored rice, quinoa, yams, or entire wheat pasta. These sources offer fundamental supplements and advance solid assimilation. Stay away from refined starches and pick entire grains whenever the situation allows.

3.   Fats: Your dog's coat, skin, and overall health require healthy fats. Incorporate fats

from sources like fish oil, flaxseed oil, or olive oil in their eating routine. These fats give omega-3 and omega-6 unsaturated fats, which support a sound-resistant framework and add to a gleaming coat. Make sure there are enough fats in your diet because too much fat can make you gain weight.

4.   Nutrients and Minerals: To keep their health at its best, dogs need a variety of vitamins and minerals. The majority of these nutrients can typically be found in a well-balanced diet, but some may require supplementation. Fundamental nutrients and minerals incorporate vitamin A, vitamin D, vitamin E, B-complex nutrients, calcium, phosphorus, zinc, and iron. A veterinarian or veterinary nutritionist can direct you on the particular necessities of your canine because of their age, breed, and any hidden medical issue.

5.   Hydration: Water is essential for your dog's health. Make sure they always have

access to clean, fresh water to drink. Dampness-rich food sources, like natively constructed stews or integrating stock into their dinners, can likewise add to their hydration.

6.   Energy Needs: The quantity of calories your canine requires relies upon different elements, including size, age, movement level, and digestion. It's critical to work out the proper caloric admission for your canine to keep a solid weight. Your veterinarian or a veterinary nutritionist can give direction on deciding the ideal day-to-day caloric admission for your canine because of their singular necessities.

Keep in mind, the healthful necessities of canines might differ, so it's critical to talk with an expert to make a customized diet plan. They can assist with surveying your canine's particular necessities, screen their well-being, and make changes depending on the situation. Normal veterinary check-ups are fundamental to guarantee that your canine remaining parts are healthy and to address any dietary worries.

Understanding your canine's nourishing necessities is vital to furnishing them with a decent natively constructed diet that advances their general well-being and bliss. You can ensure that your pet gets the nutrients they need to live a long and healthy life by carefully considering their needs and seeking professional advice.

2.2 Essential Nutrients for Dogs

To support their growth, development, and overall health, dogs require a variety of essential nutrients. While getting ready natively constructed canine food, remembering these supplements for suitable amounts is significant. The following are important dog nutrients:

1.   Protein: Since dogs are by nature carnivores, protein is an essential component of their diet. Protein gives the structure blocks to muscle improvement, tissue fixing, and the creation of chemicals and chemicals. Great creature-based proteins like chicken, meat, turkey, fish, and eggs are incredible sources. Plant-based proteins like tofu and legumes like lentils, chickpeas, and chickpeas can be used if you follow a vegetarian or vegan diet. Utilize a variety of protein sources to achieve a balanced supply of essential amino acids.

2.   Fats: Fats are a significant energy hotspot for canines and assist with keeping up with solid skin and coats. They likewise help in the assimilation of fat-solvent nutrients. Choose olive oil, fish oil, flaxseed oil, or other healthy fats. Omega-3 and omega-6 fatty acids, which support brain function, cardiovascular health, and anti-inflammatory responses, can be found

in these sources. Fats have a lot of calories, so be careful about how much you eat.

3. Carbohydrates: While canines have a restricted capacity to process carbs, they can in any case profit from them in moderate sums. In their diet, carbohydrates provide energy and fiber. Decide on complex starches like earthy-colored rice, quinoa, yams, and entire wheat pasta. These sources offer fundamental nutrients, minerals, and dietary fiber. Dogs primarily get their energy from proteins and fats, so avoid eating a lot of carbohydrates, especially refined grains, and sugars.

4. Nutrients and Minerals: Canines require a scope of nutrients and minerals to help different physical processes. Vitamins A, D, E, B-complex, calcium, phosphorus, zinc, iron, and others are among these. A well-balanced diet made up of a variety of whole foods can provide many of these nutrients. Nonetheless, a few canines might

profit from explicit enhancements or strengthened food sources. To ensure that your dog gets the vitamins and minerals it needs, talk to a vet or a veterinary nutritionist.

5.   Water: For dogs, adequate hydration is essential. Always provide your dog with clean, fresh water to drink. Dampness-rich food sources, like custom-made stews or adding water to their dinners, can likewise add to their hydration. Screen your canine's water admission and guarantee they approach water over the day.

6.   Fiber: Fiber can help regulate bowel movements and promote healthy digestion. It additionally helps with the weight of the board. Consolidate fiber-rich fixings like vegetables (e.g., carrots, green beans, pumpkin), organic products (e.g., apples, blueberries), and entire grains into your canine's dinners. Be careful not to

incorporate unreasonable measures of fiber, as it can prompt gastrointestinal bombshell.

7.   Additional Additions: Your dog may require additional supplements, such as joint support (such as glucosamine and chondroitin), probiotics for gut health, or therapeutic supplements for particular health conditions, depending on their particular requirements. Talk with your veterinarian or a veterinary nutritionist to decide whether any extra enhancements are important for your canine.

While forming hand-crafted canine food, finding some kind of harmony and meeting your canine's individual dietary needs is significant. Take into consideration speaking with a veterinarian or veterinary nutritionist who will be able to provide you with individualized advice based on the age, breed, weight, level of activity, and any underlying health conditions of your dog. Customary observing of your canine's well-being and occasional veterinary check-ups are fundamental to guarantee their wholesome prerequisites are being met actually.

2.3 Homemade vs. Commercial Dog Food

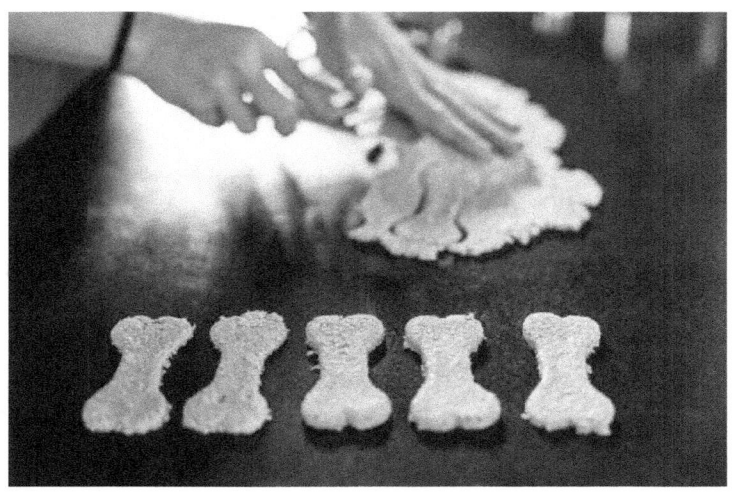

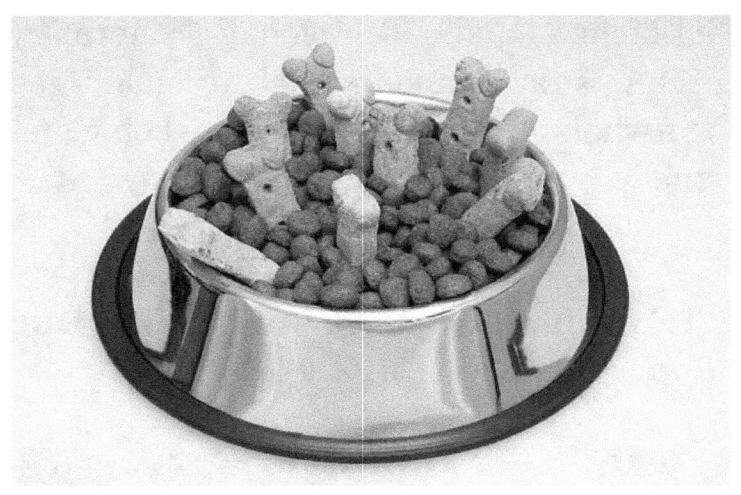

Picking among hand-crafted and business-canine food is a choice that many pet people face. The two choices enjoy their benefits and contemplations. When comparing homemade and commercial dog food, consider the following:

1. Fixing Control: With custom-made canine food, you have full command over the fixings utilized. You can select fresh, high-quality ingredients and modify the recipes to meet the particular dietary

requirements of your dog. If your dog has allergies, sensitivities, or other health conditions that necessitate a specialized diet, this level of control can be especially helpful.

2.   Quality and Wellbeing: While getting ready natively constructed canine food, you can guarantee that the fixings are of great and liberated from unsafe added substances or additives. You can pick natural, privately obtained fixings and can focus on newness and healthy benefits. Be that as it may, it's critical to deal with and store fixings appropriately to limit the gamble of pollution.

3.   Wholesome   Equilibrium: When homemade dog food is used, it can be more difficult to feed a diet that is well-balanced in nutrients. To thrive, dogs require specific amounts of vitamins, minerals, proteins, fats, carbohydrates, and other nutrients. Planning an even natively constructed diet

might require counsel with a veterinarian or veterinary nutritionist to guarantee that your canine's nourishing necessities are met. There are a lot of commercial dog foods that can be tailored to specific life stages or health conditions to provide a balanced diet.

4. Accommodation and Time Responsibility: Business canine food offers comfort since it is promptly accessible and requires negligible arrangement. Planning custom-made canine food, then again, can be tedious, particularly assuming that you decide to make huge clumps or complex recipes. Planning, shopping, cooking, and portioning are all required. In any case, a few pet people track down bliss in getting ready dinners for their fuzzy companions and consider it to be a chance for holding.

5. Cost Contemplations: Depending on several factors, homemade dog food may be less expensive or more expensive. It frequently necessitates the purchase of new

ingredients, and supplements or specialized ingredients may incur additional costs. Then again, business canine food offers a scope of choices at various price tags. Consider your spending plan and the particular healthful requirements of your canine while assessing cost contemplations.

6.   Combination and transitional feeding: Either switching to homemade food or combining the two is an option. Progressive changes permit your canine's stomach-related framework to acclimate to the new eating regimen. Consolidating business and natively constructed food can give accommodation while as yet integrating new, custom-made feasts into your canine's daily schedule.

7.   Proficient Direction: Looking for direction from a veterinarian or veterinary nutritionist is important while planning natively constructed canine food. They can assist with guaranteeing your canine's

dietary necessities are met and guide you on segment sizes, fixing choices, and any important enhancements. They can likewise screen your canine's well-being and exhort on any changes required.

Eventually, the decision between natively constructed and business canine food relies upon your canine's particular necessities, your inclinations, and your capacity to give a healthfully adjusted diet. Make an educated decision that is best suited to your dog's overall health and well-being by taking into consideration the advantages and disadvantages of each option and consulting professionals.

Chapter 3: Kitchen Essentials for Dog Food Preparation

3.1 Tools and Equipment

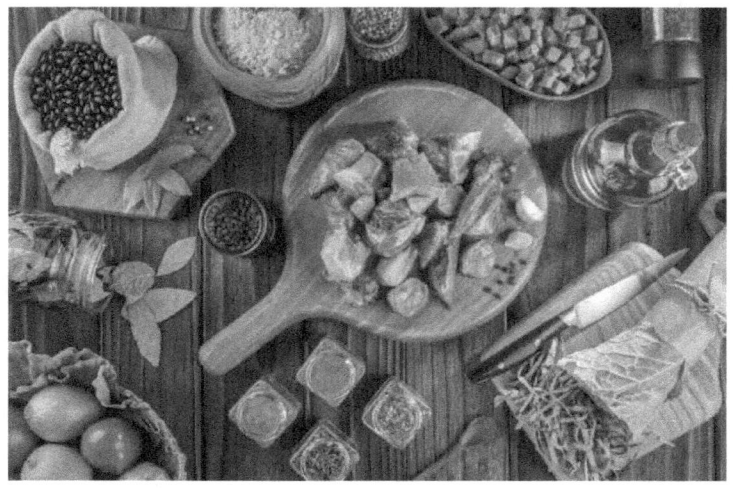

While planning custom-made canine food, having the right devices and hardware can make the cycle more productive and agreeable. Here are a few fundamental things that can help you in the readiness of handcrafted canine food:

1.   Cutting Board: A strong and clean cutting board is fundamental for cleaving and planning fixings. The ingredients you'll be working with should fit comfortably on a cutting board that is large enough.

2.   Sharp Blades: Buy a set of sharp knives that are suitable for cutting a variety of ingredients. A gourmet specialist's blade, a paring blade, and a serrated blade can cover a large portion of your cutting requirements.

3.   Dish Bowls: Have a determination of blending bowls in different sizes. This permits you to combine fixings as one and keep them coordinated during the cooking system.

4.   Estimating Instruments: Precise estimations are urgent for guaranteeing

appropriate piece sizes and wholesome equilibrium. Measure ingredients precisely with spoons and measuring cups.

5. Food Processor or Blender: For recipes that require a smooth texture or for making homemade treats, a food processor or blender can be useful for grinding or pureeing ingredients.
6. Pots and Dish: Have a scope of pots and skillets in various sizes to oblige the different recipes you'll get ready. Choose products of high quality that are easy to clean and don't stick.

7. Slow Cooker or Moment Pot: A sluggish cooker or Moment Pot can be a helpful device for getting ready hand-crafted canine food, particularly for recipes that require long, slow cooking or for group cooking.

8. Food scale: When precise measurements are required for precise

nutritional balance, a food scale lets you accurately weigh ingredients.

9. Can Opener: A dependable can opener is a necessity if you include canned ingredients in your dog's recipes.

10. Storage Facilities: For proper storage of homemade dog food, it is essential to have a supply of airtight storage containers. For easy identification and meal rotation, choose containers that are safe for food storage and label them.

11. Cooler Packs or Holders: If you intend to freeze segments of hand-crafted canine nourishment for some time later, cooler-safe packs or compartments are fundamental. They assist with keeping up with newness and forestall cooler consumption.

12. Cleaning Supplies: Keep up with great cleanliness in your kitchen by having dish

cleanser, scour brushes, and wipes for cleaning utensils, bowls, and other gear.

Make sure to clean all devices and hardware completely when use to forestall cross-pollution and guarantee the security of the food you get ready.

Having the right apparatuses and hardware can smooth out the most common way of planning hand-crafted canine food and make it more charming. Put resources into quality things that will work well for you over the long haul, and consistently focus on cleanliness and tidiness while dealing with nourishment for your fuzzy companion.

3.2 Ingredients and Shopping Tips

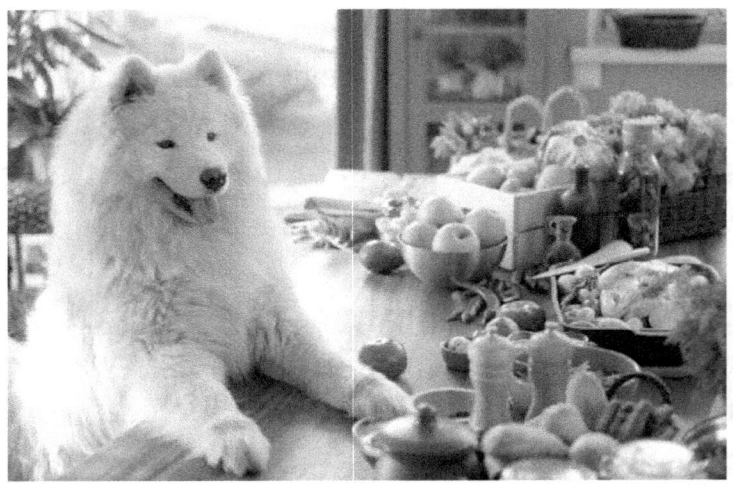

While planning natively constructed canine food, choosing the right fixings is critical to guarantee your canine gets a reasonable and nutritious eating regimen. For selecting ingredients and navigating the shopping process, consider the following suggestions:

1.   Proteins of a Higher Quality: Decide on lean, top-notch proteins as the groundwork for your canine's dinners. Pick meats like chicken, turkey, hamburger, or

fish. When possible, look for fresh, unprocessed options and organic or human-grade meats. If you're following a veggie lover or vegetarian approach, select plant-based proteins like vegetables (e.g., lentils, chickpeas) or tofu as choices.

2. New Leafy Foods: Integrate various new products of the soil into your canine's eating regimen. Carrots, green beans, peas, yams, apples, and blueberries are superb decisions. Essential vitamins, minerals, antioxidants, and dietary fiber are provided by these components. Grapes and onions, for example, are examples of certain fruits and vegetables that can be harmful to dogs.

3. Entire Grains: Entire grains like earthy colored rice, quinoa, oats, and grain can be remembered for your canine's feasts to give energy and fiber. These grains are full of nutrients and aid in digestion. White flour and rice are examples of refined grains

that lack the nutritional value of whole grains.

4.   Solid Fats: Integrate sound fats into your canine's feasts for their skin, coat, and general well-being. Omega-3 and omega-6 fatty acid sources like fish oil, flaxseed oil, or olive oil are options to consider. These fats contribute to a glossy coat and a healthy immune system. Use fats with some restraint, as exorbitant admission can prompt weight gain.

5.   Stay away from Unsafe Fixings: Dogs may be harmed or poisoned by certain human foods. Chocolate, onions, garlic, grapes, raisins, avocados, and artificial sweeteners like xylitol should be avoided. Research and get to know food varieties that ought not to be remembered for your canine's eating routine to forestall potential well-being chances.

6.   Local and organic options: Consider picking natural fixings when accessible and affordable for you. Organic alternatives may offer higher nutritional value and reduce pesticide exposure. Moreover, supporting nearby ranchers' business sectors or homesteads can give you new, privately obtained elements for your canine's feasts.

7.   Assortment and Equilibrium: To ensure that your dog eats a well-rounded diet, try to include a variety of ingredients. Incorporate various proteins, organic products, vegetables, and grains to give a scope of supplements. Assortment additionally forestalls fatigue and supports ideal well-being.

8.   Understand Marks: Read the labels carefully when purchasing commercial ingredients like canned or packaged foods. Search for choices with insignificant added substances, additives, and fake flavors. Avoid products that have a lot of fillers or

by-products and list only the essential, easily recognizable ingredients.

9. Talk with Experts: Talk with a veterinarian or a veterinary nutritionist to get explicit direction on fixing choice and dietary necessities for your canine. They can give proposals because of your canine's variety, age, weight, and particular well-being concerns.

Keep in mind, legitimate capacity and treatment of fixings are fundamental to keeping up with newness and forestalling tainting. Ingredients that are likely to spoil should be stored appropriately and following the recommended storage guidelines.

By choosing top-notch fixings and being aware of your canine's particular dietary necessities, you can make natively constructed feasts that help their general well-being and prosperity.

Chapter 4: Homemade Dog Food Guidelines

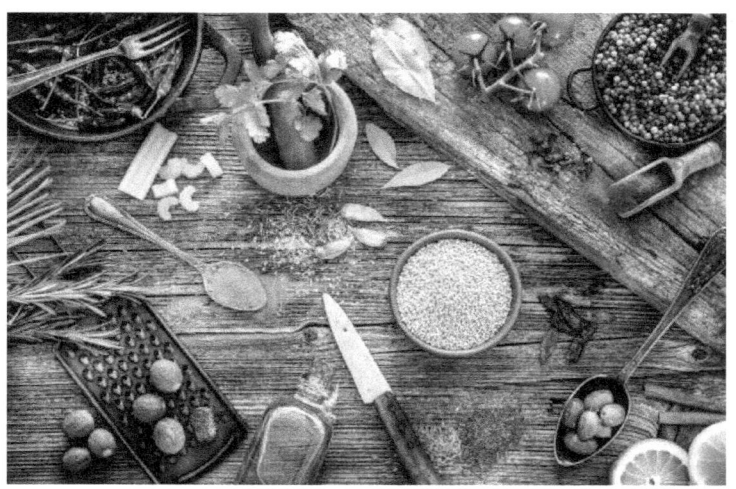

4.1 Portion Control and Feeding Guidelines

Keeping up with legitimate piece control is fundamental while planning custom-made canine food to guarantee your fuzzy companion gets the perfect proportion of nourishment without overloading or starving. Here are a few rules to assist you with laying out segment sizes and taking care of schedules:

1.   Talk with a Veterinarian: When trying to figure out how much to feed your dog, it's important to talk to a vet or a veterinary nutritionist. They can look at your dog's age, breed, weight, level of activity, and overall health to figure out what your dog needs. Your dog's nutritional needs can be met with individualized feeding guidelines from these professionals.

2.   Think about Caloric Necessities: Segment sizes ought to be founded on your canine's caloric necessities. Your dog's size, age, metabolism, and level of activity all influence the amount of calories they need. Your veterinarian can assist you in adjusting portion sizes and determining your dog's ideal caloric intake.

3.   Check your body's condition: Routinely evaluate your canine's body

condition to guarantee they are keeping a solid weight. Change segment sizes assuming that you notice weight gain or misfortune. You can evaluate your dog's overall body composition and adjust its diet accordingly with the assistance of body condition scoring systems like the 9-point scale.

4. Follow the Recipe's Directions: The recipe itself may contain guidelines for portion sizes when making homemade dog food from specific recipes. Focus on suggested serving sizes referenced in the recipe and change them given your canine's singular necessities and calorie prerequisites.

5. Consider the frequency of meals: The quantity of dinners you give each day relies upon your canine's age and inclination. Pups for the most part require more successive feasts, while grown-up canines can be taken care of a few times per day.

Isolating the everyday part into numerous feasts can assist with assimilation and forestall indulging. To determine the right amount of time your dog should eat, talk to your vet.

6. Slow Change: When switching your dog's diet from store-bought to homemade, do so gradually to allow their digestive system time to adjust. Begin by supplanting a little part of their business food with hand-crafted food, and step by step increment the extent north of up to 14 days until they are completely changed.

7. Taking care of Schedule: Lay out a steady taking care routine for your canine. Feed them simultaneously every day and in a similar area to make a feeling of routine and security. Overeating and weight gain can result from free-feeding or leaving food out all day.

8. Check your health and weight: Routinely screen your canine's weight and

general wellbeing. Monitor any progressions in their body condition, energy levels, and assimilation. If you have worries about your canine's weight or general well-being, talk with your veterinarian for additional assessment and direction.

Keep in mind that the amounts listed here are only suggestions and that every dog's needs may vary. Working intimately with a veterinarian or veterinary nutritionist will assist with guaranteeing that your canine's particular wholesome necessities are met and that their piece sizes are suitable for their age, size, and action level.

Legitimate piece control and taking care of rules are fundamental for keeping up with your canine's optimal weight, advancing their general well-being, and forestalling corpulence-related medical problems.

4.2 Transitioning to Homemade Food

To ensure a smooth adjustment, converting your dog to homemade food from commercial food should be done gradually. Here are some moves toward follow while changing your canine to a natively constructed diet:

1.   Get advice from a veterinarian: Before rolling out any huge improvements to your canine's eating regimen, talk with a veterinarian or a veterinary nutritionist. They can look at your dog's health, figure out what they need to eat, and help you transition to homemade food.

2.   Plan and study: Learn about dogs' dietary requirements and the essential nutrients they require. Research recipes and accumulate data on proper fixings and piece sizes for your canine's particular necessities.

3.   Start slowly: Start by substituting homemade food for a small amount of your dog's commercial food. For instance, you could begin by substituting homemade food for 10% of their meals and gradually increase this amount throughout one to two weeks. This permits your canine's stomach-related framework to adjust to the new eating routine and limits the gamble of gastrointestinal surprise.

4.   Screen for Stomach related Upset: Watch out for your canine during the change time frame. Watch for any indications of stomach-related upset like the runs, spewing, or changes in craving. Assuming that you notice any issues, dial back the change interaction and talk with your veterinarian.

5.   Change Part Sizes: As you increment the extent of natively constructed food in your canine's dinners, change the piece sizes to keep up with their ideal body condition

and weight. Work with your veterinarian to decide the suitable piece sizes in light of your canine's singular necessities and caloric prerequisites.

6. Survey Wellbeing and Prosperity: All through the progress, screen your canine's general well-being and prosperity. Examine their energy levels, coat condition, digestion, and any other improvements or concerns that stand out. On the off chance that you notice any medical problems or have questions, talk with your veterinarian.

7. Look for Proficient Direction: On the off chance that you're uncertain about planning a healthfully adjusted custom-made diet for your canine, think about looking for direction from a veterinary nutritionist. They can give master counsel, assist you with making a decent recipe, and guarantee your canine's particular nourishing necessities are being met.

8.   Be Patient and Adaptable: Each canine is one of a kind, and the progress cycle might differ. Be patient and adaptable, adjusting as necessary to meet your dog's specific requirements. It might require investment to find the right blend of fixings and part measures that turn out best for your canine.

Keep in mind that making the switch to homemade food is a process that needs constant monitoring and attention. By taking it step by step, looking for proficient direction, and noticing your canine's reaction, you can effectively progress them to a natively constructed diet that meets their wholesome necessities and advances their general well-being and prosperity.

Chapter 5: Meat-Based Recipes

5.1 Chicken and Rice Delight

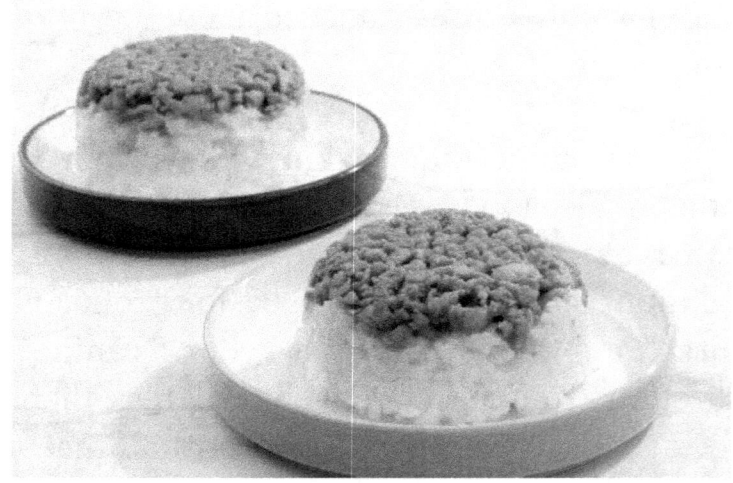

Many dogs enjoy the straightforward and nutritious Chicken and Rice Delight recipe. It contains essential nutrients, carbohydrates, and protein in a healthy balance. This recipe for homemade dog food can be made in the following manner:

Ingredients:

• 1 cup cooked and shredded boneless chicken breast
• 1 cup cooked brown rice
• 12 cups steamed or boiled mixed vegetables (such as carrots, peas, and green beans)
• 1 tablespoon olive oil Instructions:

1.   Cook the breast of the chicken: The boneless, skinless chicken breast can be cooked to perfection in a pot of water or baked. Shred the chicken into bite-sized pieces once it has been cooked. Check to see that there are no bones or skin

.

2.   Get the rice ready: Cook the earthy-colored rice as indicated by the bundle guidelines. Always cook it until it is tender and cooked all the way through. You can utilize a rice cooker or burner technique.

3.   Steam or heat the vegetables: Steam or heat the blended vegetables until they are delicate. They can be cooked in a steamer or boiling water until they are cooked but not overly soft.

4.   Join the fixings: In a blending bowl, combine as one the destroyed chicken, cooked earthy-colored rice, and steamed/bubbled vegetables. Shower the olive oil over the blend and mix well to consolidate. The olive oil gives the dish a healthy dose of good fats.

5.   Permit the blend to cool: Allow the combination to chill off before serving it to your canine. Ensure it's at room temperature or somewhat warm, as outrageous temperatures can be awkward for canines.

6.   Serve and maintain: Divide the Chicken and Rice Delight into portions that are suitable for your dog's needs and size.

Serve the meal to your dog, and any leftovers can be kept for up to three days in airtight containers in the refrigerator. You can likewise parcel individual servings and freeze them for some time in the future.

Keep in mind, segment sizes might differ relying on your canine's size, age, and action level. Talk with your veterinarian to decide the suitable serving size for your particular canine.

Lean protein, complex carbohydrates, and vegetables make up the balanced meal in the Chicken and Rice Delight recipe, which provides a variety of nutrients for your dog's overall health. Screen your canine's response to the new dinner and talk with a veterinarian if you have any worries or questions.

5.2 Beef and Sweet Potato Stew

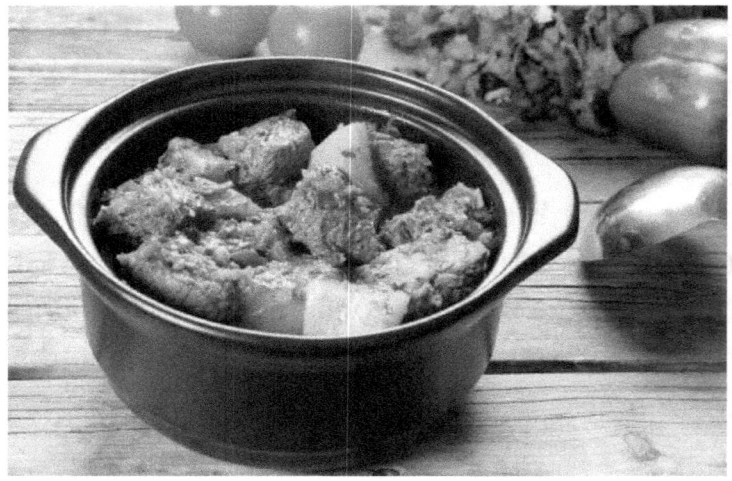

Here is a recipe for Meat and Yam Stew, a delightful and nutritious custom-made canine food choice:

Ingredients:

• 1 cup of lean ground beef
• 1 medium-sized sweet potato that has been peeled and diced
• 12 cups of fresh or frozen peas • 12 cups of diced carrots

- 1 cup of low-sodium beef or vegetable broth
- 1 tablespoon of olive oil

1. Prepare the ground beef by Lean ground beef should be cooked over medium heat until browned and thoroughly cooked in a large pot or skillet. Channel any overabundance of fat.

2. Add the vegetables: Add the diced yam, peas, and carrots to the skillet with the cooked ground meat. The vegetables should begin to soften after a few minutes of sautéing.

3. Incorporate the broth: Pour the low-sodium meat or vegetable stock into the skillet with the hamburger and vegetables. Mix well to consolidate every one of the fixings.

4. Cook and boil: Lessen the intensity to low and allow the stew to stew for around

20-25 minutes, or until the yams and carrots are delicate. Stir occasionally to ensure even cooking and prevent sticking.

5.   Sprinkle with olive oil: Not long before serving, shower the stew with olive oil. This enhances the stew's flavor and provides a healthy dose of beneficial fats.

6.   Let the stew cool down: Before serving the Beef and Sweet Potato Stew to your dog, let it cool down. Ensure it's at room temperature or somewhat warm.

7.   Serve and maintain: Divide the stew into portions that are suitable for your dog's size and requirements. Serve the feast to your canine and store any extras in sealed shut compartments in the fridge for as long as three days. You can also freeze individual servings that have been portioned out for later use.

Make sure to change segment sizes as per your canine's size, age, and action level. Talk with your veterinarian to decide the suitable serving size and address particular dietary contemplations for your canine.

The Meat and Yam Stew gives a delightful blend of lean protein from hamburger, the fiber and supplement content of yams and vegetables, and the additional hydration from the stock. It offers a balanced dinner that upholds your canine's general well-being and taste buds. Keep an eye on how your dog reacts to the new food and talk to your vet if you have any questions or concerns.

5.3 Turkey and Vegetable Medley

Here is a recipe for Turkey and Vegetable Variety, a nutritious and tasty hand-crafted canine food choice:

Ingredients:

- 1 cup lean ground turkey
- 2 cups chopped broccoli
- 2 cups chopped cauliflower
- 2 cups diced carrots
- 2 cups chopped green beans
- 1 cup low-sodium chicken or vegetable broth
- 1 tablespoon olive oil

Instructions:

1.   Prepare the ground turkey by Lean ground turkey should be cooked in a large pot or skillet over medium heat until it is fully cooked and no longer pink. While cooking, break it into small pieces. Get rid of any extra juices or fat.

2.   Add the vegetables: Along with the cooked ground turkey, add the chopped broccoli, cauliflower, carrots, green beans, and green beans to the skillet. Sauté for a

couple of moments until the vegetables start to relax.

3. Pour in the stock: Pour the low-sodium chicken or vegetable stock into the skillet with the turkey and vegetables. Mix well to consolidate every one of the fixings.

4. Stew and cook: Decrease the intensity to low and allow the variety to stew for around 15-20 minutes, or until the vegetables are delicate. Mix every so often to forestall staying and guarantee in any event, cooking.

5. Olive oil drizzled on top: Olive oil should be drizzled over the medley just before serving. This adds a sound portion of useful fats and upgrades the kind of dish.

6. Permit the mixture to cool: Permit the Turkey and Vegetable Mixture to chill off

before serving it to your canine. Ensure it's at room temperature or somewhat warm.

7. Serve and maintain: Divide the medley into portions that meet your dog's needs and size. Serve the dinner to your canine and store any extras in hermetically sealed holders in the cooler for as long as three days. You can also freeze individual servings that have been portioned out for later use.

Make sure to change segment sizes as per your canine's size, age, and movement level. Take your dog's specific dietary requirements into account and discuss the appropriate serving size with your vet.

The Turkey and Vegetable Mixture gives a nutritious mix of lean protein from turkey and an assortment of fiber-rich vegetables. Your dog's overall health and preferences will be supported by this well-balanced and flavorful option. Screen your canine's reaction to the new dinner and talk with a veterinarian on the off chance that you have any worries or questions.

Chapter 6: Fish-Based Recipes

6.1 Salmon and Quinoa Bowl

A healthy homemade dog food recipe with a lot of omega-3s is the Salmon and Quinoa Bowl:

Ingredients:

• 1 cup cooked salmon (boneless, skinless, and chipped)
• ½ cup cooked quinoa
• ½ cup peas (new or frozen)
• ½ cup carrots, diced
• ½ cup spinach, hacked
• 1 tablespoon fish oil (discretionary)

Directions:

1. Cook the salmon: Cook the salmon by baking or steaming until it is completely

cooked and effectively chips separated. Eliminate any bones or skin and chip the salmon into little, reduced-down pieces.

2.   Cook the quinoa: Follow the directions on the package to cook the quinoa. Before cooking, be sure to thoroughly rinse it. Once cooked, permit it to marginally cool.

3.   Steam or heat the peas and carrots: Peas and carrots can be cooked until tender by steaming or boiling. You can involve a liner or spot them in a pot of bubbling water. Once cooked, channel any abundant water.

4.   Combine the following: Combine the cooked salmon, cooked quinoa, peas, carrots, and chopped spinach in a mixing bowl. Make sure to thoroughly mix in all of the ingredients.

5.   Optional: Add fish oil: Fish oil can be drizzled over the salmon and quinoa

mixture if desired. Omega-3 fatty acids, which support healthy skin, coat, and overall well-being, are abundant in fish oil.

6. Permit the blend to cool: Before serving the Salmon and Quinoa Bowl to your dog, let it cool down. Ensure it's at room temperature or somewhat warm.

7. Serve and maintain: Partition the blend into fitting segments given your canine's size and needs. Serve the dinner to your canine and store any extras in hermetically sealed holders in the cooler for as long as three days. You can also freeze individual servings that have been portioned out for later use.

Make sure to change segment sizes as per your canine's size, age, and movement level. Take your dog's specific dietary requirements into account and discuss the appropriate serving size with your vet.

The Salmon and Quinoa Bowl gives a solid mix of lean protein from salmon, supplements thick quinoa, and a blend of vegetables for added nutrients and minerals. A reasonable and delightful choice backings your canine's general well-being and gives fundamental omega-3 unsaturated fats. Screen your canine's reaction to the new dinner and talk with a veterinarian on the off chance that you have any worries or questions.

6.2 Tuna and Carrot Casserole

Tuna and Carrot Casserole, a tasty and healthy homemade dog food recipe, can be found here:

Ingredients:

• 1 can of tuna in water that has been drained
• 1 cup of grated or finely chopped carrots

- 1 cup of cooked brown rice
- 2 beaten eggs
- 1 cup of low-sodium chicken or vegetable broth

Instructions:

1.   Preheat the stove: Lightly grease a casserole dish and preheat the oven to 350°F (175°C).

2.   Get the ingredients ready: In a blending bowl, consolidate the depleted fish, ground or cleaved carrots, peas, cooked earthy colored rice, beaten eggs, and low-sodium chicken or vegetable stock. Blend well to consolidate every one of the fixings completely.

3.   Move to the goulash dish: Empty the combination into the lubed goulash dish, spreading it out equally.

4.   Heat the dish: Place the goulash dish in the preheated stove and heat for around

30-35 minutes or until the meal is set and softly brilliant on top.

5. Let the casserole cool down: Eliminate the dish from the stove and permit it to cool for a couple of moments before serving it to your canine. Ensure it's at room temperature or somewhat warm.

6. Serve and store: Depending on your dog's size and requirements, divide the Tuna and Carrot Casserole into portions. Serve the meal to your dog, and any leftovers can be kept for up to three days in airtight containers in the refrigerator. You can likewise parcel individual servings and freeze them for some time in the future.

Make sure to change segment sizes as per your canine's size, age, and movement level. Talk with your veterinarian to decide the proper serving size and address particular dietary contemplations for your canine.

The tuna protein, carrots' natural sweetness and fiber, peas' additional nutrients, and the nutritious grain of brown rice in the Tuna and Carrot Casserole create a flavorful dish. A decent and fulfilling choice backings your canine's general well-being and taste inclinations. Screen your canine's reaction to the new feast and talk with a veterinarian if you have any worries or questions.

6.3 Whitefish and Spinach Chowder

Whitefish and Spinach Chowder, a tasty and healthy homemade dog food recipe, can be found here:

Ingredients:

- 1 cup whitefish filets (like cod, haddock, or sole), cooked and chopped
- 1 cup spinach, hacked
- ½ cup yams, diced
- ½ cup carrots, diced

- ½ cup low-sodium chicken or vegetable stock
- ½ cup unsweetened coconut milk

Instructions:

1. Cook the whitefish: Cook the whitefish filets by baking, steaming, or poaching until they are completely cooked and effectively piece separated. Flake the fish into bite-sized pieces by removing any skin or bones.

2. Steam or heat the yams and carrots: Sweet potatoes and carrots can be steamed or cooked in water until tender. You can steam them in a steamer or boil them in a pot of water. Once cooked, channel any overabundance of water.

3. Set up the spinach: Make small cuts in the spinach. New or frozen spinach can be utilized in this recipe.

4.   Combine the following: Steamed sweet potatoes, steamed carrots, cooked and flaked whitefish, chopped spinach, low-sodium chicken or vegetable broth, and unsweetened coconut milk should all be combined in a pot. Mix well to join every one of the fixings.

5.   Make chowder by Bringing the mixture to a gentle simmer in the pot over medium heat. It should be allowed to simmer for about ten to fifteen minutes, with occasional stirring, until the vegetables are soft and the flavors have merged.

6.   Permit the chowder to cool: Before serving the Whitefish and Spinach Chowder to your dog, let it cool down. Ensure it's at room temperature or somewhat warm.

7.   Serve and store: Partition the chowder into suitable segments in light of your canine's size and needs. Serve the meal to your dog, and any leftovers can be kept for

up to three days in airtight containers in the refrigerator. You can likewise parcel individual servings and freeze them for some time in the future.

Make sure to change segment sizes as per your canine's size, age, and movement level. Talk with your veterinarian to decide the proper serving size and address particular dietary contemplations for your canine.

Whitefish protein, spinach's high nutrient density, sweetness, and fiber from sweet potatoes and carrots make the Whitefish and Spinach Chowder a delicious meal. The coconut milk adds a smooth surface and wealth to the chowder. A balanced and delightful choice backings your canine's general well-being and taste inclinations. Screen your canine's reaction to the new feast and talk with a veterinarian if you have any worries or questions.

Chapter 7: Vegetarian and Vegan Recipes

7.1 Lentil and Brown Rice Pilaf

Here is a recipe for Lentil and Earthy colored Rice Pilaf, a nutritious and fiber-rich natively constructed canine food choice:

Ingredients:

- ½ cup earthy-colored lentils, washed
- ½ cup earthy-colored rice
- 1 cup blended vegetables (like peas, carrots, and green beans), diced
- 2 cups low-sodium vegetable stock
- 1 tablespoon olive oil

Directions:

1. Cook the lentils: In a pot, consolidate the washed lentils with 1 cup of water. After

bringing to a boil, reduce the heat to low and simmer the lentils for approximately 15 minutes, or until they are tender. Channel any overabundance of water and put it away.

2.   Cook the earthy-colored rice: In a different pot, cook the earthy-colored rice as per the bundle directions. Make a point to flush the rice completely before cooking. Put the cooked food aside.

3.   Vegetables can be boiled or steamed: Diced mixed vegetables can be cooked until tender by steaming or boiling them. You can involve a liner or spot them in a pot of bubbling water. Once cooked, channel any overabundance of water.

4.   Join the fixings: In a huge blending bowl, join the cooked lentils, cooked earthy-colored rice, and steamed blended vegetables. To fully incorporate all of the ingredients, thoroughly mix.

5.　　Shower with olive oil: Sprinkle the Lentil and Earthy-colored Rice Pilaf blend with olive oil. The pilaf's flavor is enhanced and the added oil provides beneficial fats.

6.　　Permit the pilaf to cool: Before serving the Lentil and Brown Rice Pilaf to your dog, let it cool down. Ensure it's at room temperature or somewhat warm.

7.　　Serve and store: Partition the pilaf into suitable segments given your canine's size and needs. Serve the feast to your canine and store any extras in impenetrable holders in the cooler for as long as three days. You can likewise parcel individual servings and freeze them for some time in the future.

Make sure to change segment sizes as indicated by your canine's size, age, and movement level. Talk with your veterinarian to decide the fitting serving size and address particular dietary contemplations for your canine.

The Lentil and Earthy colored Rice Pilaf gives a supplement thick mix of fiber-rich lentils and earthy-colored rice, alongside the additional nutrients and minerals from blended vegetables. A reasonable and filling choice backings your canine's general well-being and gives a decent wellspring of plant-based protein. Screen your canine's reaction to the new feast and talk with a veterinarian on the off chance that you have any worries or questions.

7.2 Chickpea and Pumpkin Stew

Here is a recipe for Chickpea and Pumpkin Stew, a nutritious and tasty custom-made canine food choice:

Ingredients:

- 1 can chickpeas, depleted and washed
- 1 cup pumpkin puree (unsweetened, canned, or cooked)
- ½ cup carrots, diced
- ½ cup peas (new or frozen)
- 1 cup low-sodium vegetable stock
- 1 tablespoon olive oil

Directions:

1.   Cook the vegetables: In a pot, consolidate the diced carrots and peas with the low-sodium vegetable stock. After bringing to a boil, reduce the heat to low and simmer the vegetables for approximately ten minutes, or until they are tender. Set aside any excess liquid after draining it.

2.   Pound the chickpeas: Use a fork or a potato masher to mash the drained and rinsed chickpeas in a bowl until they are partially mashed and some of the chickpeas are still intact.

3. Join the fixings: In a huge pot, consolidate the squashed chickpeas, pumpkin puree, and cooked vegetables. Blend well to consolidate every one of the fixings completely.

4. Turn on the stew: Stew the stew in the pot over low heat, stirring occasionally. Pumpkin can become too thick if it is boiled, so be careful not to.

5. Sprinkle with olive oil: Not long before serving, shower the Chickpea and Pumpkin Stew with olive oil. The additional oil gives solid fats and upgrades the kind of stew.

6. Permit the stew to cool: Permit the stew to chill off before serving it to your canine. Ensure it's at room temperature or somewhat warm.

7. Serve and maintain: Partition the stew into suitable bits given your canine's size and needs. Serve the dinner to your canine

and store any extras in hermetically sealed compartments in the cooler for as long as three days. You can likewise partition individual servings and freeze them for some time in the future.

Make sure to change segment sizes as indicated by your canine's size, age, and action level. Take your dog's specific dietary requirements into account and discuss the appropriate serving size with your vet.

The chickpea-based protein in the Chickpea and Pumpkin Stew is a healthy combination of pumpkin's natural sweetness and fiber, carrots and peas' additional nutrients, and chickpeas' plant-based protein. A delightful and healthy choice backings your canine's general well-being and taste inclinations. Keep an eye on how your dog reacts to the new food and talk to your vet if you have any questions or concerns.

7.3 Sweet Potato and Kale Stir-Fry

Sweet Potato and Kale Stir-Fry is a healthy and colorful homemade dog food recipe:

Ingredients:

• 1 medium-sized sweet potato, peeled and sliced thinly; 2 cups destemmed and chopped kale; 12 thinly sliced carrots; 12 fresh or frozen peas; 1 tablespoon olive oil

Instructions:
1. Sweet potatoes can be boiled or steamed: Put the sweet potato in a steamer or a pot of boiling water with thin slices on top. Cook the sweet potato until it is soft but still retains its shape. Set aside and remove any unused water.

2. Sauté the vegetables: Olive oil can be heated in a large skillet or wok over medium heat. Add the hacked kale, cut carrots, and peas. The vegetables should be slightly

softened after 5-7 minutes of sautéing, with occasional stirring.

3.   Add the yam: Steamed sweet potato slices should be gently added to the skillet with the sautéed vegetables. Mix well to consolidate every one of the fixings.

4.   Pan sear: Stir-frying the mixture for another 3 to 5 minutes until the kale is wilted and the sweet potatoes are heated through. Be mindful so as not to overcook the vegetables, as they ought to in any case hold some surface.

5.   Let the stir-fry cool down: Permit the Yam and Kale Sautéed food to chill off before serving it to your canine. Make sure it is either slightly warm or at room temperature.

6.   Serve and store: Depending on your dog's size and requirements, divide the stir-fry into appropriate portions. Serve the

feast to your canine and store any extras in sealed shut compartments in the fridge for as long as three days. Make sure to parcel individual servings and freeze them for some time in the future whenever wanted.

Keep in mind to adjust portion sizes based on your dog's age, size, and level of activity. Talk with your veterinarian to decide the suitable serving size and address particular dietary contemplations for your canine.

The Yam and Kale Pan fried food gives a nutritious mix of fiber-rich yams, salad greens from kale, and the additional nutrients and minerals from carrots and peas. It is a vibrant and healthy option that is good for your dog's overall health and tastes. Screen your canine's reaction to the new dinner and talk with a veterinarian if you have any worries or questions.

Chapter 8: Treats and Snacks

8.1 Peanut Butter Banana Biscuits

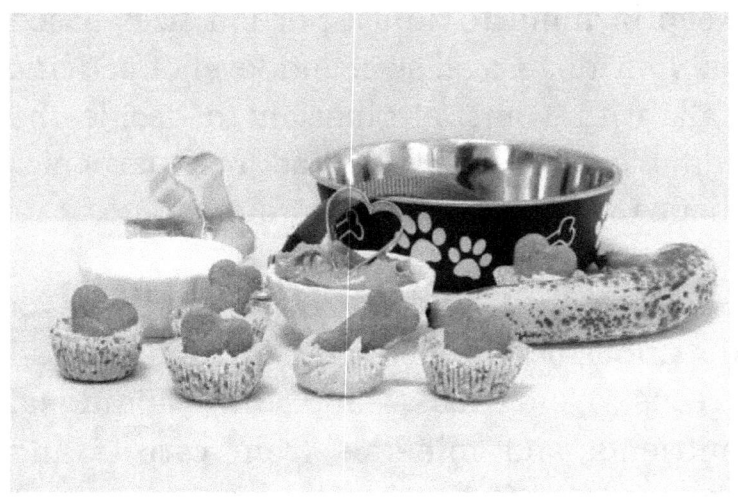

Here is a recipe for Peanut Butter Banana Rolls, a tasty and natively constructed canine treat choice:

Ingredients:

- 2 ready bananas, crushed
- ½ cup regular peanut butter (ensure it doesn't contain xylitol)
- 1 ½ cups entire wheat flour
- 1 teaspoon baking powder

Directions:

1. Get the oven ready: Prepare a baking sheet by lining it with parchment paper and preheating the oven to 350°F (175°C).

2. Blend the wet fixings: In a blending bowl, consolidate the squashed bananas and peanut butter. Blend well until they are consolidated.

3. Add the dry fixings: To the banana and peanut butter mixture, add the baking powder and whole wheat flour. Mix well until a batter structures. You can add a little more flour if the dough is too sticky.

4.   Carry out the mixture: On a gently floured surface, carry out the mixture to about ¼-inch thickness. A rolling pin can be used to get an even thickness.

5.   Remove the rolls: Utilizing a cutout or a blade, cut out roll shapes from the moved batter. You can make small, bite-sized biscuits or choose shapes that your dog likes.

6.   Put the bread rolls on the baking sheet: Move the slice-out bread rolls to the pre-arranged baking sheet, leaving a touch of room between every bread roll.

7.   Heat the rolls: Bake the baking sheet for about 15-20 minutes, or until the biscuits are golden brown and firm to the touch. Place the baking sheet in the preheated oven.

8.   Cool and store: Eliminate the baking sheet from the broiler and let the rolls cool

totally on a wire rack. The Peanut Butter Banana Biscuits should be kept at room temperature once they have cooled. They can be kept for up to two weeks in storage.

Keep in mind to adjust the biscuit portion sizes based on your dog's size, age, and dietary requirements. As part of a healthy diet, these treats should be enjoyed in moderation.

The Peanut Butter Banana Bread rolls are a delicious and healthy treat for your canine, consolidating the regular pleasantness of bananas with the overpowering kind of peanut butter. They make an extraordinary prize or nibble choice that your fuzzy companion will cherish. Make these homemade biscuits for your beloved pet with pleasure!

8.2 Carrot and Apple Pupcakes

Carrot and Apple Pupcakes, a healthy homemade treat for your dog, can be found here:

Ingredients:

- 1 ½ cups entire wheat flour
- 1 teaspoon baking powder
- ½ teaspoon cinnamon (discretionary)
- 1 cup ground carrots
- 1 medium-sized apple, stripped and ground
- 2 tablespoons honey
- 2 eggs
- ½ cup unsweetened fruit purée
- ¼ cup water

Guidelines:

1.   Preheat the broiler: Prepare a muffin pan by lining it with paper liners and preheat the oven to 350°F (175°C).

2.   Blend the dry fixings: In a blending bowl, join the entire wheat flour, baking powder, and cinnamon (if utilized). The dry ingredients should be thoroughly mixed in.

3.   Add the ground carrots and apple: Add the ground carrots and ground apple to the dry-fixing combination. Blend well to disseminate the carrots and apples uniformly.

4.   Combine the wet components: Whisk the applesauce, water, honey, and eggs in a separate bowl until well combined.

5.   Mix the dry and wet ingredients: Empty the wet fixing combination into the bowl with the dry fixings. Mix until every one of the fixings is completely integrated and a thick player structure.

6.   Fill the biscuit tin: Spoon the player equally into the paper liners in the biscuit tin, filling everyone around 66% full.

7.   Prepare the cupcakes: Place the biscuit tin in the preheated stove and prepare for roughly 18-20 minutes, or until the cupcakes are firm and brilliant brown on top.

8.   Serve once cooled: The cupcakes should cool completely on a wire rack after being removed from the oven. When they have cooled, you can give them to your dog as a tasty and nutritious treat.

Keep in mind to alter the cupcake portion sizes following your dog's age, size, and dietary requirements. These cupcakes are intended to be given with some restraint as a component of a fair eating regimen.

Combining the natural sweetness and fiber of carrots and apples with the wholesomeness of whole wheat flour, the Carrot and Apple Pupcakes are a flavorful and wholesome treat for your dog. They make a unique treat for birthday events, festivities, or just to show your shaggy companion some additional affection. Appreciate making these natively constructed cupcakes for your cherished little guy!

8.3 Pumpkin Spice Bites

Here is a recipe for Pumpkin Zest Nibbles, a wonderful and occasional custom-made canine treat choice:

Ingredients:

- 2 cups moved oats
- ½ cup pumpkin puree (unsweetened, canned, or cooked)
- ¼ cup unsweetened fruit purée
- 2 tablespoons honey
- 1 teaspoon cinnamon
- ½ teaspoon ground ginger
- ¼ teaspoon ground nutmeg

Directions:

1.   Preheat the broiler: Preheat your broiler to 350°F (175°C) and line a baking sheet with material paper.

2.   Combine the oats: In a food processor or blender, beat the moved oats until they structure a coarse flour-like consistency. Place aside.

3.   Blend the wet fixings: In a blending bowl, consolidate the pumpkin puree, unsweetened fruit purée, honey, cinnamon, ground ginger, and ground nutmeg. Mix well to consolidate the wet fixings completely.

4.   Add the oat mixture: Blend the oats and gradually add them to the wet ingredient mixture. Give it a thorough stir until the ingredients are fully incorporated and the dough is thick.

5. Shape the chomps: Roll small amounts of the dough into bite-sized balls. The size can be changed to suit your dog's preference.

6. Put on the baking sheet: Organize the molded pumpkin flavor chomps on the pre-arranged baking sheet, leaving a touch of room between everyone.

7. Heat the nibbles: Place the baking sheet in the preheated stove and heat for roughly 15-18 minutes, or until the chomps are firm and gently brilliant.

8. Cool and serve: Eliminate the baking sheet from the broiler and let the pumpkin zest nibbles cool totally on a wire rack. You can give them to your dog as a tasty holiday treat once they have cooled.

Make sure to change the part sizes of the pumpkin flavor chomps as indicated by your canine's size, age, and dietary necessities. As part of a healthy diet, these treats should be enjoyed in moderation.

The Pumpkin Zest Nibbles are a delectable and merry treat for your canine, consolidating the kinds of pumpkin, cinnamon, ginger, and nutmeg. They make a magnificent occasional treat or whenever bite that your shaggy companion will appreciate. Make these homemade treats for your beloved dog with fun!

Chapter 9: Special Diets and Health Concerns

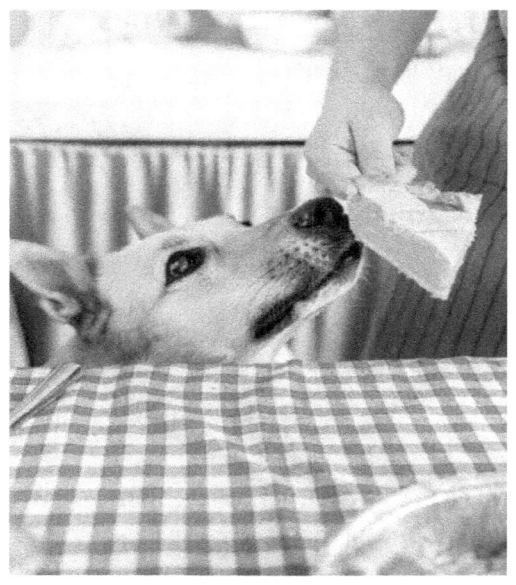

9.1 Grain-Free Recipes

The following are three sans-grain recipes for canines:

1. *Sans grain Chicken and Yam Stew:*

Ingredients:
- 1 cup sliced boneless, skinless chicken breast
- 1 cup peeled and diced sweet potatoes
- 12 cup chopped green beans
- 12 cup diced carrots
- 1 cup low-sodium chicken broth
- 1 tablespoon coconut oil

Instructions:

1. In an enormous pot, heat coconut oil over medium intensity.

2. Add the diced chicken bosom and cook until caramelized and cooked through.

3. Add the yams, green beans, carrots, and chicken stock to the pot.

4. Heat the blend to the point of boiling, then, at that point, diminish the intensity and stew for around 20 minutes or until the vegetables are delicate.

5.   Before serving the stew to your dog, let it cool.

6.   Serve in portions that are suitable for your dog's size and requirements.

7.   Without grain Meat and Vegetable

2. Pan fried food:
Ingredients:

- 1 cup lean ground hamburger
- ½ cup broccoli florets, slashed
- ½ cup cauliflower florets, slashed
- ½ cup ringer peppers, diced
- 1 tablespoon coconut aminos (a soy sauce elective)
- 1 tablespoon olive oil

Instructions:
1.   In an enormous skillet or wok, heat olive oil over medium intensity.

2.   Add the lean ground meat and cook until caramelized and cooked through.

3.   Add the broccoli, cauliflower, and chime peppers to the skillet and sautéed food for around 5 minutes or until the vegetables are fresh and delicate.

4.   Sprinkle the coconut aminos over the sautéed food and mix to cover the fixings.

5.   Permit the pan-fried food to cool before serving it to your canine.

6.   Serve in suitable bits because of your canine's size and needs.

7.   Sans grain Salmon and Zucchini

3. Cakes:
Ingredients:

•	1 can wild-caught salmon, depleted and chipped
•	1 cup zucchini, ground and abundance dampness pressed out
•	1 egg
•	½ cup almond flour
•	1 tablespoon coconut oil

Directions:

1.	In a blending bowl, join the chipped salmon, ground zucchini, egg, and almond flour. Make sure to thoroughly mix everything.

2.	Make tiny patties out of the mixture.

3.	Heat coconut oil in a skillet over medium heat.

4. Cook the salmon and zucchini cakes for around 3-4 minutes on each side or until they are brilliant brown and cooked through.

5. Permit the cakes to cool before serving them to your canine.

6. Serve in fitting bits in light of your canine's size and needs.

Make sure to change segment sizes as indicated by your canine's size, age, and movement level. It is always a good idea to talk to your veterinarian about the right serving size and any special dietary requirements your dog may have. Appreciate setting up these without-grain recipes for your furry companion!

9.2 Weight Management Meals

The following are three dog weight management meal ideas:

1. *Medley of Lean Turkey and Vegetables:*

Ingredients:

- 1 cup lean ground turkey
- ½ cup carrots, diced
- ½ cup green beans, cleaved
- ½ cup peas (new or frozen)
- 1 tablespoon olive oil

Instructions:

1.   In an enormous skillet, cook the hung ground turkey over medium intensity until completely cooked. Get rid of any extra fat.

2.   Add the diced carrots, hacked green beans, and peas to the skillet with the cooked turkey. Sauté the vegetables for a few minutes until they are tender.

3. Sprinkle the blend with olive oil for added sound fats.

4. Permit the feast to cool before serving it to your canine.

5. Serve in suitable parts in light of your canine's size and weight the executives' objectives.

2. Mash fish and sweet potatoes: Ingredients:

• 1 cup cooked and flaked white fish filets (such as cod or haddock)
• 1 cup cooked and mashed sweet potatoes
• 12 cups green peas (fresh or frozen)

Instructions:

1. Cook the white fish filets by baking, steaming, or poaching until completely

cooked. Eliminate any bones or skin and drop the fish into little pieces.

2.   Mash the sweet potatoes after cooking them until tender.

3.   Cook the green peas until delicate.

4.   Flaked fish, mashed sweet potatoes, and cooked green peas should be combined in a mixing bowl. Mix thoroughly until all of the ingredients are distributed evenly.

5.   Before serving the mash to your dog, let it cool.
6.   Serve in proper bits in light of your canine's size and weight of the executives' objectives.

3.   Chicken and Broccoli Sautéed food:

Ingredients:

- 1 cup boneless, skinless chicken bosom, diced
- 1 cup broccoli florets, slashed
- ½ cup carrots, meagerly cut
- 1 tablespoon coconut aminos (a soy sauce elective)
- 1 tablespoon olive oil

Instructions:

1. Olive oil can be heated in a large skillet or wok over medium heat.

2. Add the diced chicken bosom and cook until sautéed and cooked through.

3. Add the hacked broccoli and daintily-cut carrots to the skillet. Pan-sear for around 5 minutes or until the vegetables are fresh and delicate.

4. Toss the stir-fry with the coconut aminos and stir to coat the ingredients.

5. Permit the pan-fried food to cool before serving it to your canine.

6. Serve in portions that are appropriate for your dog's size and weight control goals.

Make sure to change segment sizes as per your canine's size, progress in years, and endlessly weigh the board objectives. It's in every case best to talk with your veterinarian to decide the suitable serving size and address particular dietary contemplations for your canine's weight the board needs

9.3 Allergies and Sensitivities

With regards to sensitivities and awareness in canines, it's critical to distinguish and stay away from explicit allergens that can set off unfriendly responses. The following are a couple of contemplations for overseeing sensitivities and responsive qualities in canines:

1. Determine the allergens by Working with your veterinarian to recognize the particular allergens causing your canine's responses. Normal allergens incorporate specific proteins (like hamburgers, chicken, or dairy), grains (like wheat or corn), and natural variables (like dust or residue vermin).

2. Disposal diet: Assuming that food sensitivities are thought of, your veterinarian might suggest a disposal diet. This involves feeding your dog a diet with only a few ingredients that include novel sources of protein (like duck or venison) and carbohydrates that are easy to digest (like sweet potatoes or peas). Continuously acquaint new fixings with pinpoint any unfavorably susceptible responses.

3. Diets free of allergens: Monetarily accessible hypoallergenic diets can likewise be a possibility for overseeing sensitivities. These eating regimens utilize hydrolyzed proteins or novel protein and carb sources to limit the probability of setting off hypersensitive responses.

4. Diets made at home: On the off chance that your canine has numerous sensitivities or responsive qualities, your veterinarian might suggest a painstakingly formed hand-crafted diet. This guarantees total and adjusted nourishment while keeping away from explicit allergens.

5. Evasion of natural allergens: Reduce exposure if your dog has allergies to the environment. This might incorporate limiting open air time during high dust seasons, keeping your home clean and residue-free, and utilizing air channels or purifiers.

6.   Treats with few ingredients: Pick treats made especially for dogs who have sensitivities or allergies. Search for choices that utilize elective protein and starch sources, keeping away from normal allergens like wheat, corn, and soy.

7.   Daily grooming: Grooming your dog regularly can help remove allergens from its skin and coat. Brush your dog's coat to get rid of any potential irritants and bathe them with hypoallergenic shampoos that your veterinarian recommends.

8.   Talk with a veterinarian: Continuously talk with your veterinarian for a legitimate finding and direction on dealing with your canine's sensitivities or responsive qualities. They can make recommendations that are specific to you and, if necessary, they can give you medications to help you feel better.

Keep in mind that tailored approaches based on your dog's particular requirements are necessary for managing allergies and sensitivities in dogs. Normal correspondence with your veterinarian is significant for deciding the best strategy and guaranteeing your canine's prosperity.

Chapter 10: Tips for Meal Prep and Storage

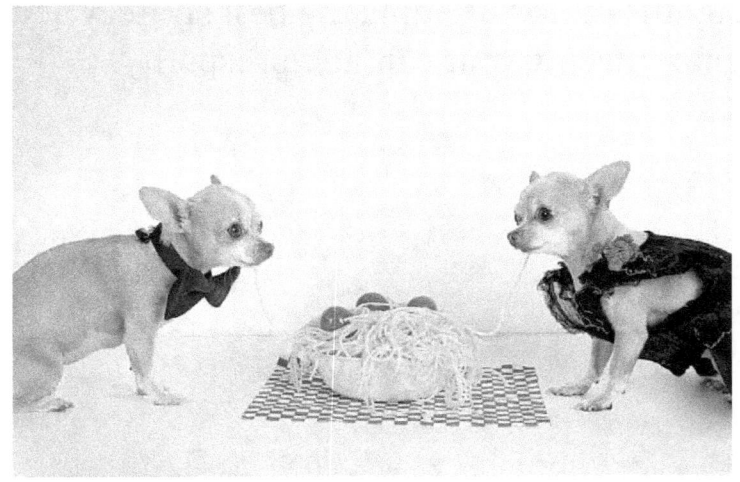

10.1 Batch Cooking and Freezing

A quick and easy way to make sure your dog always has access to homemade, healthy food is to cook meals in bulk and freeze them. For batch cooking and freezing dog meals, follow these guidelines:

1.   Plan your dinners: Choose your recipes in advance and the quantities you want to prepare. Take into account your

dog's dietary requirements, portion sizes, and any particular ingredients or restrictions.

2. Assemble fixings: Make a shopping rundown and assemble every one of the fundamental elements for your chosen recipes. Guarantee you have appropriate capacity compartments or cooler sacks for putting away the feasts.

3. Cook in mass: Get ready bigger clusters of canine feasts than you would for a solitary serving. This enables you to save as much time and effort as possible while ensuring that multiple meals are prepared for freezing.

4. Segment control: Partition the prepared dinners into individual segments given your canine's size, age, and dietary necessities. Use estimating cups or a kitchen scale to guarantee precise part measures.

5.   Refresh the meals: Before packaging the cooked meals for freezing, let them cool completely. This aids in the prevention of bacterial growth and excessive moisture.

6.   Choose the right containers for storage: Utilize water/airproof holders or cooler safe packs to store the feasts. Mark every compartment with the name of the recipe and the date of the groundwork for simple distinguishing proof.

7.   Freeze the feasts: To save space, place the portioned meals in the freezer, ensuring that they are stored flat. Before sealing, remove any excess air from freezer bags. Guarantee the cooler temperature is set at 0°F (- 18°C) or beneath to keep up with food quality and forestall deterioration.

8.   Defrosting and warming: At this point when now is the right time to serve a frozen dinner, defrost it in the cooler short-term or utilize the thaw-out setting on your

microwave. Before serving, slightly warm the meal but not too hot for your dog. Abstain from defrosting and refreezing a similar feast more than once to keep up with food handling.

9.   Revolution and newness: Utilize a turn framework to guarantee dinners are consumed in a sensible time. Consume the most established frozen feasts first and recharge your cooler stock with new clumps routinely to keep up with quality and healthy benefits.

10.   Obtain advice from your veterinarian: Regarding portion sizes, particular dietary requirements, and any potential concerns or considerations for your dog's diet, always consult your veterinarian.

By bunch-preparing and freezing canine dinners, you can save time, guarantee a reliable stockpile of quality food, and have the comfort of prepared-to-serve feasts at whatever point is required. It's an incredible method for giving your canine adjusted and nutritious natively constructed food while keeping up with newness and quality.

10.2 Proper Food Storage Practices

Legitimate food stockpiling rehearses are fundamental for keeping up with the newness, quality, and well-being of your canine's food. Here are a few rules to keep while putting away canine food:

1.   Store in a cool, dry spot: Pick a capacity region that is cool, dry, and away from direct daylight. Heat and humidity can speed up the deterioration of food and increase the risk of spoilage.

2.   Keep it sealed: Make certain that dog food is kept in resealable bags or airtight

containers made specifically for pet food storage. This helps keep pests, moisture, and air from affecting the quality of the food.

3. Utilize unique bundling or move appropriately: Assuming that you like to keep food in its unique bundling, ensure it's firmly fixed after each utilization. On the other hand, move the food to a reasonably sealed shut holder, guaranteeing it is spotless and dry before adding the food.

4. Check for damage or tears: Consistently examine the bundling or compartments for any tears or harm that could think twice about food's newness or draw in brothers. Supplant-harmed bundling or compartments depending on the situation.

5. Keep in mind when they run out: Focus on the "best by" or termination dates on the canine food bundling. To ensure that

you are feeding your dog the freshest food possible, use the oldest packages first.

6.   Stay away from cross-defilement: On the off chance that you have numerous kinds of canine food or treats, keep them put away independently to forestall cross-defilement of flavors or possible allergens. If your dog has particular dietary requirements or allergies, this is especially crucial.

7.   Try not to blend old and new food: While adding another pack or bunch of food, make an effort not to blend it in with the remainder of the old food. This keeps up with consistency and forestalls possible issues with old or ruined food.

8.   Clean utensils and feeding bowls: Routinely spotless and clean your canine taking care of bowls, scoops, and utensils to forestall the development of microbes or

defilement. Use soapy, hot water to thoroughly rinse.

9. Think about freezing or refrigerating: Assuming you get ready for natively constructed canine food or buy new/frozen choices, adhere to explicit capacity directions. Quickly freeze or refrigerate perishables to preserve their quality and stop the growth of bacteria.

10. Talk with your veterinarian: Assuming you have explicit different kinds of feedback about appropriate food stockpiling rehearses for your canine's eating regimen, talk with your veterinarian. They can give direction in light of your canine's particular necessities and dietary prerequisites.

You can aid in preserving the nutritional value, freshness, and safety of your dog's food by adhering to these recommended food storage practices. It's memorable's vital that various kinds of canine food might have explicit capacity proposals, so consistently allude to the bundling or talk with the maker for a particular direction.

Chapter 11: Frequently Asked Questions

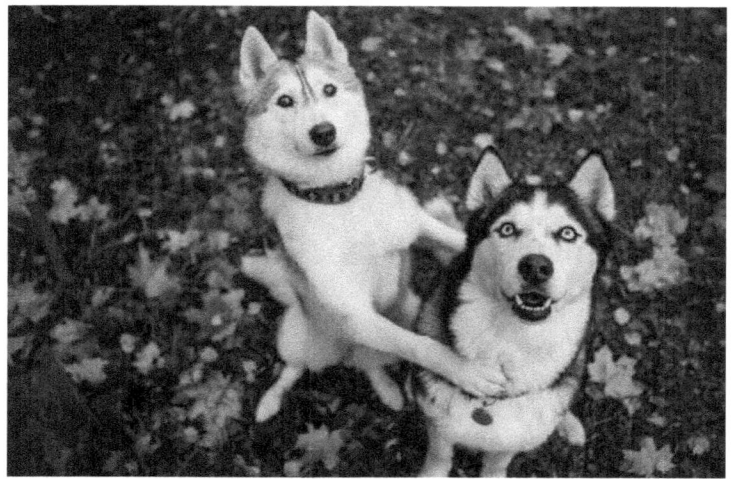

11.1 Can I supplement commercial food with homemade meals?

As long as you adhere to the following guidelines and take into consideration, it is generally safe to supplement your dog's commercial food with homemade meals:

1.   Talk with your veterinarian: It's important to talk to your vet before making any changes to your dog's diet. They can

give direction in light of your canine's particular necessities, ailments, and dietary prerequisites.

2.   Keep things in balance and eat well: Guarantee that any custom-made feasts you plan give a fair and complete wholesome profile for your canine. This incorporates suitable measures of protein, starches, solid fats, nutrients, and minerals. Consider talking with a veterinary nutritionist to make even natively constructed recipes or utilize laid-out recipes from legitimate sources.

3.   Comprehend segment sizes: Decide the suitable part estimates for your canine in light of their size, age, movement level, and any weight the board objectives. Remember that hand-crafted feasts might have different caloric densities contrasted with business food varieties, so segment sizes might be changed likewise.

4. Change over time: Assuming you choose to enhance business food with hand-crafted feasts, acquaintance with the new food steadily will permit your canine's stomach-related framework to change. Start with a small amount of the homemade meal, then gradually increase it over a few days.

5. Screen your canine's reaction: Notice your canine's response to the new eating routine. Search for any indications of stomach related agitation, like loose bowels, regurgitating, or changes in craving. Screen their weight and in general wellbeing to guarantee they are blossoming with the joined eating regimen.

6. Assortment and pivot: Giving different food varieties can assist with guaranteeing a more extensive scope of supplements. Pivot the fixings in your natively constructed feasts and differ the recipes over the long haul to keep supplement lacks or awarenesses from creating.

7.	Safety and quality: Use high-quality ingredients like fresh vegetables, lean proteins, and whole grains (if they're included). To reduce the likelihood of bacterial contamination, ensure proper food handling, storage, and hygiene practices.

8.	Keep the base of commercial food: While hand-crafted dinners can be a sound expansion, keeping a great business canine food as the foundation of your canine's diet is by and large suggested. Commercial foods undergo stringent testing and quality control to meet the nutritional requirements of dogs.

Keep in mind, each canine is remarkable, and their dietary prerequisites might shift. The best source for individualized advice tailored to your dog's needs is your veterinarian. They can assist you with making a reasonable and reasonable eating regimen that consolidates business food with natively constructed feasts to guarantee your canine's ideal well-being and nourishment.

11.2 What ingredients should I avoid feeding my dog?

Due to their potential to harm or be toxic to dogs, several ingredients should not be fed to your dog. Here are a few critical fixings to keep away from:

1.   Chocolate: Chocolate contains theobromine and caffeine, which are harmful to canines. These chemicals can be more harmful in higher concentrations in dark chocolate and cocoa powder. Indeed, even limited quantities of chocolate can cause side effects like regurgitation, loose bowels, fast breathing, expanded pulse, and even seizures.

2.   Raisins and grapes: Dogs can develop kidney failure from raisins and grapes. Due

to the unknown toxic compound, grapes and raisins should not be given to your dog at all.

3.   Onions and garlic: Onions and garlic contain intensities that can harm a canine's red platelets, prompting frailty. These fixings are especially harmful when consumed in enormous amounts or over a drawn-out period.

4.   Xylitol: Xylitol is a sugar-free artificial sweetener that can be found in a variety of sugar-free confections, gum, and baked goods. Xylitol can cause a fast arrival of insulin in canines, prompting a perilous drop in glucose levels. It can bring about side effects like a shortcoming, heaving, seizures, and, surprisingly, liver disappointment.

5.   Avocado: Avocado contains persin, a compound that can be harmful to canines in enormous sums. While the tissue of ready

avocados is for the most part ok for canines in little amounts, the pits, skin, and leaves can be harmful and represent a gagging peril.

6.   Alcohol: Dogs are extremely toxic to alcohol. Even a small amount can cause severe symptoms like vomiting, diarrhea, problems with coordination, depression of the central nervous system, and, in extreme cases, respiratory distress or coma.

7.   Caffeine: Caffeine, found in espresso, tea, caffeinated drinks, and certain soft drinks, can be risky for canines. It may result in restlessness, rapid breathing, an elevated heart rate, tremors, and seizures that are analogous to chocolate poisoning.

8.   Bones: Cooked bones can fragment and make stifling perils or interior wounds canines. Instead of giving your dog cooked bones, especially poultry bones, choose safer options like dental chews made with special

ingredients or raw bones that your veterinarian recommends.

9. High-salt food sources: Dogs can become dehydrated and have electrolyte imbalances if they consume too much salt. Try not to take care of your canine high-salt food sources like pungent bites, handled food sources, or food varieties prepared with a ton of salt.

10. Certain nuts: Macadamia nuts, for example, can be toxic to dogs and cause weakness, tremors, vomiting, and hyperthermia.

It's vital to take note that this rundown isn't comprehensive, and there might be different fixings that can be destructive to canines. Continuously talk with your veterinarian on the off chance that you have any different kinds of feedback about unambiguous food varieties or fixings to guarantee you are giving a protected and suitable eating regimen for your shaggy companion.

11.3 How can I ensure a balanced diet for my dog?

Guaranteeing a decent eating regimen for your canine is significant for their general well-being and prosperity. Here are a few hints to assist you with giving a healthfully adjusted diet to your canine:

1.   Talk with your veterinarian: Look for direction from your veterinarian to decide your canine's particular healthful necessities. Factors, for example, age, size, breed, movement level, and any ailments ought to be considered while arranging their eating routine.

2.   Select commercial dog food of high quality: Select a business canine food that is named "complete and adjusted" or

"healthfully complete." Search for items that fulfill the nourishing guidelines set by perceived associations, for example, the Relationship of American Feed Control Authorities (AAFCO).

3. Peruse the fixing list: Focus on the fixings recorded on the canine food bundling. Search for genuine meat sources (like chicken, hamburger, or fish) as the essential fixing. Keep away from food sources that contain fake additives, varieties, or flavors.

4. Observe taking care of rules: Follow the feeding instructions on the packaging of the dog food. These rules regularly propose suitable piece sizes given your canine's weight. Change the piece sizes as important to keep a sound load for your canine.

5. Give various proteins: Integrate an assortment of protein sources into your canine's eating routine. Lean meats, fish,

poultry, and plant-based proteins like lentils or chickpeas are examples of this. Offering different protein sources guarantees your canine gets a scope of fundamental amino acids.

6. Include vegetables and fruits: Add products of the soil to your canine's eating routine as a wellspring of nutrients, minerals, and fiber. Carrots, sweet potatoes, blueberries, apples, and green beans are all suitable alternatives. Make sure to stay away from poisonous food varieties like grapes, raisins, onions, and garlic (as examined in a past reaction).

7. Limit your intake of sweets: Limit the number of treats you give your canine to forestall overloading and supplement irregular characteristics. Treats ought to just make up a little part of their day-to-day calorie consumption. Settle on sound, low-calorie treats or utilize little bits of standard food as remunerations.

8. Think about dietary enhancements: You may want to consider including dietary supplements in your dog's diet after consulting with your veterinarian. Supplements like omega-3 unsaturated fats or joint wellbeing enhancements can be helpful for specific canines. Nonetheless, consistently counsel your veterinarian before presenting any enhancements.

9. Keep an eye on your dog's health and weight: Consistently screen your canine's weight and body condition. Change their piece estimates or talk with your veterinarian assuming you notice critical weight gain or misfortune. It is essential to have your pet examined by a veterinarian regularly to evaluate their overall health and talk about any dietary changes.

10. Be aware of changes: Make gradual changes to your dog's diet if you decide to do so. Present new food varieties or diet

changes gradually over a time of a few days to permit their stomach-related framework to change.

Keep in mind that every dog is different and has different nutritional requirements. Your veterinarian is the best asset to give customized counsel and direction to guarantee your canine's eating regimen is adjusted and custom-made to their particular requirements.

Chapter 12: Conclusion and Final Thoughts

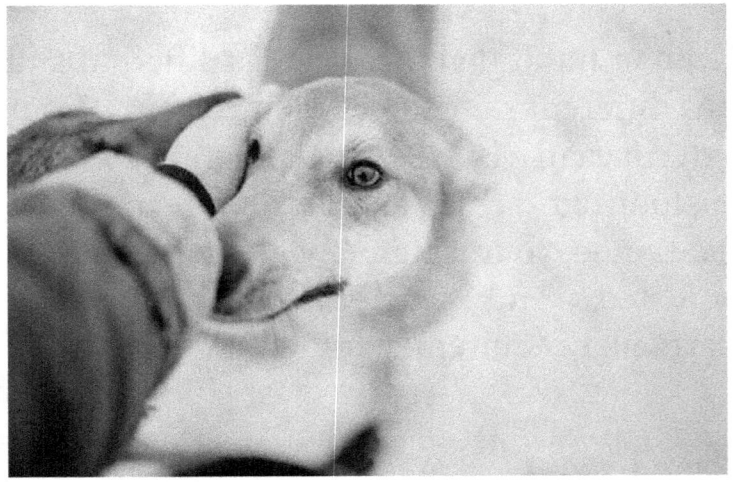

All in all, giving an even and nutritious eating regimen is essential for your canine's general well-being and satisfaction. You can ensure that your dog receives the necessary nutrients, maintains a healthy weight, and avoids harmful ingredients by adhering to the guidelines discussed in this conversation. Talking with your veterinarian is constantly prescribed to address particular dietary necessities or worries for your canine.

Whether you pick business canine food, custom-made feasts, or a mix of both, it's vital to focus on quality fixings, segment control, and assortment. Your dog's diet should be well-balanced, stored appropriately, and regularly checked for weight and overall health.

Keep in mind that different dogs may have particular health issues or dietary requirements that necessitate specialized care. Your veterinarian is your best asset for customized guidance in light of your canine's particular requirements.

In conclusion, giving affection, care, and thoughtfulness regarding your canine's healthful necessities remains closely connected with their general consideration. Building a sound and adjusted diet for your dearest pet will add to their drawn-out well-being and joy.

Continuously keep an open line of correspondence with your veterinarian, remain informed about the most recent examination and rules, and partake in the excursion of sustaining your canine with nutritious feasts. Your pet will live a vibrant and fulfilling life thanks to your dedication to their diet.

* 9 7 9 8 8 5 2 5 5 0 5 3 8 *